The Gout Book

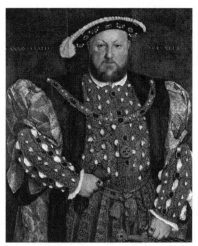

Gout is a royal pain.
Henry VIII suffered from it.

Gout is a man's disease, occurring seven to nine times more often in men than women. It's also a common disease, striking an estimated 3.4 million American men annually. That makes gout the most prevalent form of inflammatory arthritis in men older than 40.

The Harvard Medical School Family Health Guide [1]

Men in their 40s and 50s are most likely to develop gout. But by age 60, gout affects men and women roughly equally. After age 80 more women than men have gout.

Arthritis Today

Disclaimer

The author is not a medical doctor, nor has he any formal training in this field. The contents of this book are not intended as a practice of medicine, but rather as a reference for sufferers of gout so that they may ask their own physicians more pertinent and informed questions. The author encourages all gout sufferers, without exception, to heed their physician's advice and to base all treatment decisions on that advice.

None of the information contained herein is intended to replace or contradict the advice and care provided by the reader's physician. In any instance of conflict, where the information in this book may seem contrary to the information being provided by a physician, the information being provided by a licensed physician takes absolute precedence. Please bring related questions to the attention of your physician, and do not act upon any information in this book without first consulting your physician.

The author is not responsible for any consequences of any actions taken by readers, whether or not they also consult their physicians. If the reader does not accept that, then please do not read further.

Introduction

At the time of writing, I am a 52-year-old Caucasian male wearing one brand new sneaker that has the front half removed. That's because my normally size-13 left foot is so swollen that it won't physically fit into a size 14 EEE shoe. The only way that I can get around with some modicum of comfort is to wear these crazy guy shoes, and if people make jokes about them, I just don't care.

Gout, as you already know, is no joke. The pain is debilitating, voracious, mood altering, extreme and invasive. Its impact affects the entire family, and sometimes co-workers and friends, because it renders a grown man helpless – unable to walk, drive, climb stairs, sometimes even dress himself. Showering can be quite an adventure. Small grandchildren become offensive missiles in the vicinity of the affected foot.

For many gout sufferers, drugs like indomethacin can calm an attack, and allopurinol helps avoid future events. Diet helps, too, as do exercise and weight control. But for an alarming number of victims, the drugs either don't work as expected, or they have side effects that create more problems. For example, I can't use indomethacin because it causes internal bleeding.

This book is intended to describe the nature of gout, its causes and symptoms, list the triggers that bring on new attacks, and explain the treatment options. There are low purine shopping lists that you can take to the grocery store, and use in the kitchen.

My goal is to help you avoid cutting off the front halves of your shoes. Dads are already the targets of so much cruel family humor: why should we give those horrible kids any more ammunition?

Table of Contents

Chapter 1
Diet and Genes: the Causes of Gout

Most gout sufferers already know that the disease is the result of an accumulation of uric acid crystals in the joints. But that simple explanation raises more questions than it answers. Knowing the causes of gout can radically increase our understanding of how the enemy thinks, and in turn can help us predict his maneuvers and prepare a defense.

There is no hard and fast cure for gout, but we can most certainly deal with it in a way that will minimize and even eliminate attacks. The key is to figure out what's happening during an attack. And the first thing we know is that people who suffer from gout usually have abnormally high levels of uric acid.

What is uric acid?

According to the US Institutes of Health [2], uric acid is "a chemical created when the body breaks down substances called purines. Most uric acid dissolves and travels to the kidneys, where it passes out in urine. If your body produces too much uric acid or doesn't remove enough if it, you can get sick. A high level of uric acid in the body is called **hyperuricemia**".

Normal uric acid values range between 3.5 and 7.2 mg/dL, and this can be determined with a simple blood test. People suffering an attack can have levels of 10, even 12 mg/dL or higher. But not all elevated test results mean that the patient has gout.

The cause could also be one (or several) of the following: acidosis, alcoholism, chemotherapy-related side effects, diabetes, excessive exercise, hypoparathyroidism, lead poisoning, leukemia, nephrolithiasis, polycythemia vera, a purine-rich diet, renal failure, toxemia related to pregnancy, and many other problems. The point is that it doesn't pay to assume that one has gout.

Only a doctor can confirm it.

There is also a noteworthy anomaly that, during an attack, some patients actually test with lower than normal levels of uric acid. The current thinking is that this happens because many of those problem cells are so busy causing havoc in your toe that they don't have time to appear in blood being extracted elsewhere for testing.

How does one develop high uric acid levels?

Doctors at the Mayo Clinic [3] have determined that high uric acid levels can be caused by either overproduction of uric acid in the body, or by decreased elimination of uric acid in the urine (or both). Specifically, factors that may cause high uric acid concentration in one's blood include genetics and diet, and also diuretic medications (water gain pills), excessive alcohol or caffeine consumption, Hodgkin's lymphoma (Hodgkin's disease), underactive thyroid, leukemia, Niacin (vitamin B-3), non-Hodgkin's lymphoma, obesity, psoriasis and some immune-suppressing drugs.

A purine-rich diet contributes somewhat, but perhaps not as much as one might think. Genetics and/or other health issues account for most high uric acid.

While there is a common perception in the general population that gout sufferers cause their own pain through a rich diet, that simply isn't true. The body produces almost all of our purines internally. The main direct source of purines is not food, but food is definitely a contributing factor. It can be the straw that breaks the camel's back, raising uric acid levels beyond the tipping point and instigating an attack.

Gout is a slow process, often taking decades to build up, and years of eating high purine foods can contribute to that. This is why suddenly changing one's diet won't instantly cure gout.

Before going on a low-purine diet, you need to discuss your plans with your physician. Changing eating habits during, or just after, a gout attack can actually trigger another one. And keep in mind that the problem begins in the kidneys, so your doctor may have some advice about avoiding related problems too, such as renal diseases and kidney stones.

What are purines?

Mosby's Medical Dictionary [4] defines purines as "any one of a large group of nitrogenous compounds. Purines are produced as end products in the digestion of certain proteins in the diet, but some are synthesized in the body. Purines are also present in many medications and other substances, including caffeine, theophylline (a drug used to relieve symptoms in respiratory diseases such as COPD and asthma), and various diuretics, muscle relaxants, and myocardial stimulants. **Hyperuricemia** (high uric acid) may develop in some people as a result of an inability to metabolize and excrete purines. A low-purine diet or a purine-free diet may be required. Foods that are high in purines include anchovies and sardines; sweetbreads, liver, kidneys, and other organ meats; legumes; and poultry. The foods lowest in purine content include eggs, fruit, cheese, nuts, sugar, gelatin, and vegetables other than legumes."

The George Mateljan Foundation sponsors a Web site called "The World's Healthiest Foods" [5]. The Foundation is a not-for-profit entity with no commercial interests or advertising, and it defines purines as:

"Natural substances found in all of the body's cells, and in virtually all foods. The reason for their widespread occurrence is simple: purines provide part of the chemical structure of our genes and the genes of plants and animals. A relatively small number of foods, however, contain concentrated amounts of purines.

For the most part, high-purine foods are also high-protein, and they include organ meats like kidney, fish like mackerel, herring, sardines and mussels, and also yeast.

"When cells die and get recycled, the purines in their genetic material also get broken down. Uric acid is the chemical formed when purines have been broken down completely. It's normal and healthy for uric acid to be formed in the body from the breakdown of purines. In our blood, for example, uric acid serves as an antioxidant and helps prevent damage to our blood vessel linings, so a continual supply of uric acid is important for protecting our blood vessels."

The Gale Encyclopedia of Medicine says that a purine is "a white crystalline substance that is one of the building blocks of DNA", while the American Heritage® Medical Dictionary says they are a "colorless crystalline organic base that is the parent compound of various biologically important derivatives". I'm sure they're both right, but this is an example of how confusing all of the information on gout can be to a patient. It often contradicts itself, especially in the area of trying to determine which foods are low in purines, or which drug therapies have the fewest side effects (see the relevant chapters for answers to both). The bottom line for gout sufferers is that purines are something that makes unwelcome levels of acid in our bodies, and when that turns to crystals that lodge in our joints, they can make a grown man cry. Been there.

Why does gout hurt so much?

So far, we've seen that purines are among the building blocks of DNA, that they are sometimes found in food, and that they're mostly created in the body. As purines are processed by the body after cells die, they become uric acid. When too much uric acid accumulates, uric acid crystals (called **monosodium urate crystals**) can become deposited in our tendons, joints, kidneys, and other organs. This is gout (gouty arthritis).

Those crystals hurt because they are shaped like sewing needles, long and thin with sharp points on the ends. Kidney stones, which are related, also have a sharp, crystalline shape that tears at the walls of organs, and thus cause pain.

Dr. S. A. Schumacher of the Achilles Foot Health Centre in Surrey, BC, Canada[6] says that gout attacks "tend to occur in the cooler parts of the body, and in areas where there is relatively more trauma, so the foot is the most common location of gout attacks. While the classic example of gout is the great toe joint, it is commonly seen in the heels, ankles, knees, and around joint capsules, tendons and other structures, too. Gout can occur in the arms and hands too, though much less frequently. In chronic cases, you may also see deposits of uric acid crystals known as tophi, or tophaceous deposits (singular is tophus), in other parts of the body, like the ears and nose, though because there is no joint, these deposits tend not to hurt. They may be visible underneath the skin, and when removed, look a lot like feta cheese."

Dr. Schumacher's point is that gout can appear almost anywhere in the body, but that it hurts most in the joints, especially those in the foot.

Joints, like the moving parts of an engine, require lubrication. In the big toe, the knee and other joints, this lubricant is known as synovial fluid. It has the consistency of a raw egg (as in "ovum", the Latin for egg, which is part of its name), and it reduces friction between moving areas of cartilage. This fluid is where those crystals reside.

During the day, most of us move about and the synovial fluid is in motion. That helps to keep crystals from settling in the joint. During sleep (or long evenings sitting on a La-Z-Boy® watching television), this is no longer true, and that accounts for much of the reason that gout most often attacks during the night. Those crystals also like it a bit cooler when they're turning from acid to crystals (fluid to solid), and the big toe is just about as far as they can get from the heart. And, of course, we have developed a culture that eats our heaviest meal (and usually the one containing the most purines) not too long before we go to bed.

As these sharp, needle-shaped crystals settle in the joint, they cause irritation, which quickly turns to inflammation.

Reacting to that, chemicals from white blood cells (plasma and leukocytes) stream to the site to combat what they perceive as an infection, which of course increases the amount of disturbing activity. They are trying to rid the body of foreign matter. So, not only are there sharp little pins sticking into the cartilage and the area surrounding the synovial sac, but the white blood cells in your body are at war with what they think is an infection, and the friendly fire takes its toll. The increased blood flow leads to redness and warmth, and some fluids leak into neighboring tissue, causing swelling. All of this activity works together to stimulate nerves, which of course results in pain. The response by our bodies is actually an immune system process, and as such it can vary widely depending on one's general health and fitness.

Traditions

Historically, gout was known as a rich man's disease. It seemed that an inordinate number of the "upper class" suffered from it, most commonly men above forty. There are no definitive historical studies, but anecdotal evidence seems to support the assumption.

Some of the reasons may indeed be related to lifestyle and class culture. For example, workingmen habitually drank large quantities of liquids (water in the fields, milk at home, even beer in the tavern), which would tend to flush one's system and help remove uric acids. Richer men drank more concentrated alcohol (spirits and wines), so the volume of liquid they consumed and expelled may well have been quite a bit lower than that of their employees. Rich men also spent more time in offices and drawing rooms than in fields or factories, so they were often more corpulent (okay, fat). Weight and exercise are both factors in gout.

Purine-rich diets may also have had some effect on the aristocracy. While most of the population in Europe and America ate a fairly constant, unremarkable and repetitive menu (lots of potatoes and bread), wealthy families often routinely dined on bacon, sweetmeats, kidneys, shellfish, legumes and other foods high in purines.

The combination of low fluid intake, low levels of exercise and a high purine diet would definitely create an environment that is hospitable to gout triggers. Remarkably, the tables have turned. Today, people at the lower end of the economic scale tend to eat fewer fresh vegetables and more processed meats. And we are all more sedentary, thanks to cars, televisions and computers.

Which brings up an uncomfortable but essential truth.

Walking helps avoid gout.

Chapter 2
Gout Symptoms

Gout symptoms are pretty wide-ranging, and can often be confusing. That is, you may have symptoms that look and feel like gout, but they could actually be something else. The only way to definitively diagnose gout is to have your doctor stick a needle in the affected joint, withdraw some of the fluids and look for crystals of uric acid. The very thought of doing that, in the middle of an attack, is horrific.

Rather than going that route, doctors normally use what a lawyer might call circumstantial evidence to identify gout. They diagnose it by identifying its symptoms and eliminating other possibilities. If there is any doubt in your doctor's mind, he/she will confirm their diagnosis with a simple blood test that reveals the level of uric acid in a patient's blood. Typically, someone suffering an attack will have elevated levels (during my last attack it was 12 mg/dL, while the recommended level to avoid attacks is less than 6 mg/dL). Normal values range between 3.5 and 7 mg/dL. Unfortunately, a few people actually show normal uric acid levels during an attack, so the blood test isn't definitive on its own.

Even if you have suffered several attacks and are so familiar with the disease that you are completely convinced the current one is gout, it is still imperative that you have your doctor confirm it. Gout presents in a way that can often be indicative of other more serious, related diseases, which can sometimes be obscured or disguised by gout.

Self-diagnosis can cause you to ignore something that may be more detrimental in the long run.

Don't assume that you have gout. Get it checked.

Gout symptoms may include:

• Sharp, extremely sensitive pain at the tip of the big toe (the most common).

• Arthritic-type intermittent pain in the joint where the big toe meets the foot (it comes and goes and feels like bone rubbing on bone). This often appears when we are squatting a lot, such as when putting on the golf course, or working on low objects that require us to "sit on our heels".

• Pulsing pain (rather than a steady stream) in the big toe, which lasts for several minutes and then goes away. Sometimes this can be lessened a bit by moving the foot, elevating it, or even rubbing it if it isn't too sensitive.

• A tired, low level, long-lasting pain in the big toe joint that feels like your shoes are too stiff, or too tight. Wearing steel-toed boots can exasperate this.

• Inflamed skin over the sesamoid bone (the bulge on the inside of your foot where the big toe starts), and this is often accompanied by mild pain.

• Swollen, aching feet. This can often be due to bad shoes, standing on concrete all day at work, or other simple causes.

• Shin pain. This can present as a sharp point of pain in the front of the leg halfway between the ankle and the knee. Runners often have shin splints that are similar, and other medical conditions including cardiac problems can also result in this kind of pain, which is definitely a reason to visit your doctor. If shin pain shows up during or immediately after a gout attack that was in the foot/ankle, it may be a symptom of gout.

• Tender knees that are sensitive to the slightest touch
• Pain along the outside of the foot.
• Swelling of an ankle, or of both.
• Pain in an ankle similar to a sprain: if you don't remember injuring or twisting your ankle, gout may be the culprit.
• Sharp, arthritic-like pain in other joints including the elbows, wrists and fingers. Quite often, these are caused by something other than gout (usually a different type of arthritis), but it's still a possibility.
• Tenderness in a joint.
• Warm skin over a joint, along with swelling.
• As the pain recedes, the skin over a joint may start to peel.
• Discoloration (red to purple) around a joint.
• Restricted movement in a joint (often aggravated by pain and sensitivity).
• Inflammation of the burse sacs in the elbow or knee.

Once again, let me stress that **it is absolutely essential that you visit with your doctor,** explain your symptoms, and let him/her diagnose whether or not you have gout. Many of the symptoms listed above can also be attributed to rheumatoid arthritis, osteoarthritis, or even a bacterial infection. Vague symptoms such as swollen, aching feet can be evidence of everything from cheap shoes to congestive heart failure.

Beyond the fact that self-diagnosis can lead us to believe that something else is gout, one of the most worrisome aspects of this disease is that, untreated (or treated improperly), it can become so many things.

Untreated, gout can lead to joint deterioration and other problems. The most obvious one is recurrent attacks, which usually develop into a pattern called chronic gout, or chronic gouty arthritis. This often ends up presenting as deformed joints (knurly growths on the big toe, finger knuckles, etc.), and these may physically inhibit motion. It becomes difficult to walk, grasp objects, turn pages, or even drive, especially with a manual transmission where the clutch needs to be depressed. Chronic gout also brings a lot of pain with it.

If chronic gout is left untreated, as it often is in countries without an advanced healthcare system, it can advance to the point that patients develop cottage cheese-like growths under the skin (the tophi mentioned earlier). These are actually crystals of uric acid, and the most common places they show up are on the ear, fingers or toes, and in some cases near the ankle, knee or elbow. Onset is usually several years after the first signs of gout. Tophi are malleable when new (that is, they're soft enough to move around), but as they develop into white nodules and then minor masses, they can become disfiguring and, typical of gout, quite painful. They eat into both bone and cartilage, and can misalign joints so that fingers and toes no longer point straight. Tophi can also increase uric acid levels in the body, contributing to a cyclical elevation of gout symptoms.

The only solution is to reduce uric acid levels in the body, and this can be done through a combination of diet and drug therapies. (You'll find more information on this in the relevant chapters.)

Chapter 3
Things That Trigger An Attack

A visit from your mother-in-law can bring on gout! Read on...

We're not always able to identify the exact moment when uric acid levels rise high enough to bring on a gout attack, but there are several known triggers. Many researchers believe that stress is one of them. Teenagers who are being teenagers, bills and budgets, an evil boss, or even houseguests (your mother-in-law) can raise one's stress level. Whether that's a direct trigger for gout, or just sets the stage for other behaviors that initiate an attack (increased use of alcohol, for example), is still being studied.

Arthritis Today [7], a publication of the Arthritis Foundation, lists the following gout triggers:

• Joint injury. (Physical stress on a joint that results in a sprain, torn ligament or even a fracture can galvanize the white blood cells into a reaction that, if uric crystals are present, will cause an attack of gout.)

• Surgery or sudden, severe illness.

• Taking certain diuretic medications for high blood pressure, leg swelling (edema), or heart failure.

• Chemotherapy.

• Starting a uric acid-lowering treatment.

• Taking the drug cyclosporine.

• Infection.

• Crash diets and fasting.

- Eating foods high in purines.
- Dehydration.
- Drinking too much alcohol.
- Drinking sweet sodas.

The magazine doesn't mention that stress can also be a contributing factor, as can sedentary habits where the legs get little exercise. Long evenings watching television with elevated feet allow crystals to accumulate in the lower joints. And emotional stress, as it does in so very many ways, can cross the line from a mental to a physical problem. Fortunately, both of these conditions can be relieved by moderate exercise. Walking for thirty minutes each evening can literally transform one's life. Using a treadmill is a substitute, as is swimming or biking, but a simple walk is really all that we need.

One of the Foundation's triggers is "eating foods high in purines". These include red meats, organ meats and most fowl. They also include lots of seafood (salmon, shrimp, mussels, crab, trout, mackerel, anchovies, scallops and sardines), and even some vegetables such as mushrooms, cooked spinach, cauliflower, peas, asparagus and lentils. (For a complete list, see Chapter 7.) Avoid alcohol, caffeine, fried food, baked goods, ice cream and rich desserts – saturated fats and sugars can increase uric acid levels, and impair kidney function.

On a more positive note, gout patients can eat cheese (low-fat), milk, eggs and most fruits and vegetables, plus many cereal and bread products.

Most of us should drink four to six 12-oz bottles of water (or the equivalent) a day, to help flush uric acid from their bodies. However, if one has other medical problems that involve water retention, this is not a good idea. Check with your doctor before making any changes to your regular diet or exercise habits.

At the other end of that spectrum, drinking too little water (dehydration) is a known gout trigger that can also bring on kidney stones. If you think gout pain is horrific, wait until you pass a large stone. One woman we spoke with says it's like giving birth to a Volkswagen - with the doors open!

I spent eleven hours on a Christmas Eve some years ago in the emergency room of a hospital in Dublin, Ireland, bent double with the most excruciating pain imaginable, which the doctor attributed to a kidney stone. We had flown across the Atlantic in midwinter and the cabin of the plane was extremely dry. Unfortunately, I didn't realize how much moisture one loses in an eight-hour flight at thirty thousand feet with the cabin heat full on.

But here's another one of those conflicting gout messages. While dry conditions and dehydration are most definitely triggers, the New York Times [8] reported in 2006 that "hot and humid weather may also be strongly associated with recurrent gout attacks". Their report was based on a paper presented at the American College of Rheumatology's Annual Scientific Meeting that year. "Such weather," the Times said, "can cause sweating and, ultimately, dehydration, which has long been recognized as a potential trigger for gout attacks."

Well, maybe that's not so conflicting after all. Temperature and dew point (but not rainfall) were factors.

And the article concluded, rather sensibly, that "drinking more water and fluids when it's warm outside could help persons with gout prevent future attacks."

Too rigorous a workout, or one that's simply too strenuous for one's physical conditioning, can be a problem. Long summer hikes for couch potatoes can trigger gout, as can dance classes, soccer and similar workouts. But golf, swimming and above all, walking within reason are highly recommended.

At the 2010 meeting of the American College of Rheumatology, Tuhina Neogi, MD, PhD, an associate professor of medicine at Boston University School of Medicine, presented a paper with preliminary findings that indicated that caffeine is a gout trigger. In a study of over 600 gout patients, Neogi's team discovered that, as the number of servings of caffeinated beverages increased, so too did the chance of having recurrent gout attacks. However, there was once more a mixed message from the gods of gout. People who regularly drank several cups of coffee a day showed little inclination toward gout attacks when their quota was increased, but people who usually didn't use caffeine showed a rather remarkable susceptibility to attack when they consumed two or more beverages a day. While the team didn't draw an irrefutable link between caffeine and gout attacks, they certainly raised enough questions to make one think twice about ordering that third Espresso Con Panna at Starbuck's™.

Some medical conditions increase one's risk of contracting gout, including diabetes and pre-diabetes, high levels of cholesterol and triglycerides, obesity (primarily in the stomach area), and high blood pressure. While not triggers themselves, they create an environment where triggers are more effective. That is, it can take less for a gout attack to develop when these conditions are present. But don't over-react to a few pounds of belly-fat. Extreme dieting will actually INCREASE uric acid levels in the blood, contributing to the factors that cause gout.

On the other hand, as the nation becomes fatter, the number of gout cases has skyrocketed. A high-calorie intake along with love handles will increase the level of uric acid in the blood, and decrease the efficiency of the kidneys. High triglyceride levels have the same effect. Getting one's weight under control in a reasonable manner, and under a doctor's guidance, is really the first step toward eliminating gout attacks.

The Arthritis Foundation is a national not-for-profit organization that provides knowledge and support to sufferers of more than a hundred different types of arthritis, including gout. It has been around since 1948, and has already funded more than $380 million in research grants! It also provides public health education, weighs in on public policy and legislation, and conducts "evidence-based programs to improve the quality of life for those living with arthritis".

Beer is a big trigger. Wine apparently is not.

Traditionally, people have believed that wine was a major cause of gout, and a trigger. However, accumulated alcohol in the system is a trigger, so while wine in moderation probably won't induce an attack, an excess may. There is some evidence that red wine has more potential than white to cause problems.

Diuretic drugs (used to rid the body of excess fluids, such as those gathering in the ankles of patients with cardiovascular problems) are a gout trigger. Unfortunately, they lower the level of fluid traveling through the kidneys, reducing their ability to rid the body of excess uric acid.

Allopurinol, the most prescribed medication for gout, can also be a trigger. In most cases, once it has been used for a while, it is not. But for new patients, it is not uncommon for Allopurinol to actually trigger a flare-up.

People with organ transplants, especially heart patients, are susceptible to gout, and one of the medications they use, cyclosporine, is a potential trigger.

In rare cases, bacterial infections can bring about a gout attack, as can minor injuries. A stubbed toe, twisted ankle, even a distended thumb can be cause for uric acid crystals to accumulate in a joint.

High doses of aspirin can trigger an episode of gout, as can levodopa and the vitamin, niacin. Levadopa is prescribed for Parkinson's disease.

If you suffer from gout, or have a loved one who does, the Arthritis Foundation is your ally. If you wish to help continue and expand the fight against gout, there are several ways that you can become involved with the Foundation.

Whether you become a member, make a donation or remember them in your will, your contribution goes to support cutting-edge research and scientifically proven programs designed to help people with arthritis.

For every dollar donated to the Foundation, more than 76 cents goes directly to fund research and activities for people afflicted with arthritis, many of whom also have mothers-in-law.

Chapter 4
Coping With An Attack

When gout strikes, there are a number of things we can do to lessen its impact on our bodies, our families and our lives. The first of these is obvious: make a doctor's appointment as soon as the first signs show up. Every hour counts. Catching gout in its earliest stages means that the meds have a smaller battle to fight. Most of the drug therapies start working rather quickly, so the sooner they are introduced, the sooner you'll feel better.

Gout can drag down the most optimistic personalities. The constant pain wears on us and eventually we succumb to grumpiness and self-pity. Our inclination, and indeed most medical advice, is to lie down with the foot elevated, and pretty much give in.

My personal experience has been that a proactive attitude is healthier. I find ways to deal with the pain and discomfort, and try in every way possible to carry on with normal life. My work involves spending some time on my feet in the workshop and some at a desk. On bad days, I don't stay home. I just spend more hours at the desk, sometimes with my foot on a stool. Keeping busy keeps my mind off the pain.

At home, nothing makes me happier than having my four little grandchildren underfoot. When the gout is especially bad, my first instinct is to wish they would stay home and leave me in peace. But once they arrive, I find within minutes they completely extract me from the self-absorbed cocoon I have erected.

Before I know it, tears of laughter have replaced the tears of pain.

Sure, it's hard to move about. We obviously can't go jogging, but we can still manage to get in the car, go to the park, sit on a bench and enjoy a little sunshine.

Keeping up one's spirits is imperative when living with pain. We simply can't afford to let it win. There will be slumps, times when all we want to do is remain immobile and scream inside, but most of the time gout pain is quite bearable and we need to get over ourselves and get on with life. The enemy is just a little tiny crystal. We can kick his butt.

Dealing with pain

The big toe is gout's favorite target. Extreme sensibility in the joint or tip of the toe can be excruciating. Until the meds kick in, the best way to deal with this in bed is to prop up a pillow on either side of the foot and allow the bed sheet to form a tent above the toe, so that the sheet doesn't actually touch it. Sometimes, two pillows on either side are needed.

If possible, have your bed partner sleep in another room, or move yourself to the spare room or even the couch, when the attack is especially severe. No matter how gentle and caring they try to be, they're going to cause some movement that will result in a brief but intensely painful episode for you.

If the foot or toe is very painful but not yet swollen, don't try heat on it unless your doctor specifically recommends it. If there is swelling and redness, an ice pack can help reduce the inflammation, but check with your doctor first. Some medications (such as ibuprofen) seek out the physically hottest part of the body and go to work there, so ice may be counterintuitive.

Heat is pretty much never a good idea during a gout attack. While the crystals are still forming they like a cool environment, which is one reason they choose a spot so far away from your body's internal furnace. Keeping your feet warm at night when there is no sign of the disease may be a good idea. But, once inflamed, the joint should be kept cool until it heals, and the temperature recedes.

Keep your full weight off the foot, even if you can bear it. This doesn't mean that one should lie down and elevate it for several days. I use a cane (walking stick), so that I don't put all of my 6 foot 2 inch (decidedly un-slim!) body weight on an affected toe, foot or ankle every time I take a step. If the left foot is affected, I hold the cane in my right hand. It helps to spread the body weight between the sore foot and the cane. If the cane is on the same side as the sore foot, I tend to lean that way and put more weight on the foot.

Make sure the cane has a rubber foot. Sticks harvested from trees in the back yard are fine, but without a rubber foot, they can be deadly on a lot of surfaces. If you trust your balance to a cane that doesn't have traction, you'll go down.

Crutches are a better solution than a cane because they transfer all the work to the arms and shoulders, and one can actually keep the sore foot completely off the ground. Most pharmacies and medical supply stores will rent crutches at extremely reasonable rates, or they'll sell them for less than the cost of a tank of gas. Crutches are definitely cumbersome and they attract unwanted attention, but they make us functional.

Rest often. Keep active, but don't overdo it.

One of the problems with gout is that it interferes with one's natural gait (using crutches or not), and something called compensation pain comes into play. This means that other muscles, joints and ligaments are doing the work that your affected limb normally does, and pretty soon the other leg/foot/ankle/hip starts to hurt, too. Even the arms that carry your weight on crutches can hurt, along with shoulders, back and buttocks. There's no sense in swapping one problem for another.

If compensation pain becomes a problem, it's not okay to add some over-the-counter pain remedy to the drugs that your doctor prescribed.

If you're taking a non-steroidal anti-inflammatory (NSAID) for gout pain, and you add ibuprofen, you can cause bleeding in colon fissures, hemorrhoids and other areas. That's because these drugs do a lot of the same things, so you are in effect overdosing. This will appear as blood in the stool. Before self-medicating, call the doc.

Back in college, I took a course in marketing. The instructor kept pounding on the concept that "perception is reality". What he meant was that it often doesn't matter what is actually true: what matters is what people believe is true. There are a lot of holes in that argument, but it does carry some truth. The public in general believes that gout is self-inflicted, so don't expect a lot of sympathy. You can talk about kidneys and purine processing until the cows come home, and everyone will nod politely and agree with you, but in their evil little hearts they still believe that you just ate too many donuts.

When your feet swell, you can take an old pair of shoes and cut off the front halves from the laces to the toes, leaving the soles in place. Old shoes work a lot better than going out and buying new sandals. The insoles are already formed to your feet, and after the attack subsides, you have a great excuse to go shopping. Make sure the unsupported sole doesn't cause new problems by catching on things and tripping you up, or by getting stuck under a pedal in the car. It may be necessary to trim the sole, too, to avoid these events. If your right foot is affected, it is probably not safe to drive a car with an automatic transmission, as you may not be able to put adequate pressure on the brake pedal. If you drive a stick shift, either foot being affected pretty much eliminates safe driving because you need to depress both the clutch and the brake pedals.

Most medications, especially narcotic pain ones, also impair your ability to drive because they cause short periods of inattentiveness, and they can induce sleep at the wheel. If public transport isn't an option, maybe it's time for a sick day.

Many of the medications for gout seem to have a mild diuretic effect. That is, they tend to make us urinate a little more frequently than usual. If you're experiencing this, and it's causing some concern, be assured that it's normal. This effect seems especially true of some painkillers.

It can actually be a good thing, because it forces us to get up off the recliner several times in the evening and go to the bathroom. Moving your body keeps fluids flowing through the affected areas, and as long as it's not causing undue stress, even this slight amount of exercise helps the immune system deal with gout.

That diuretic action expels fluids, and they must be replenished or one can dehydrate. Check with your doctor before changing your habits, but in general it's a good idea to drink a lot of water when gout attacks. Drinks with sugar and caffeine are not a good idea. Whole fruit juices are recommended, but not the ones that say cocktail or punch. The best idea is to add just enough of the whole juice to water to make it palatable. That is, seriously dilute the juice. The idea is to make water tasty, so that you drink enough water and not too much sugar. When you're not being active, your body doesn't need any extra complex sugars.

You'll probably notice that the color of your urine is a little more pronounced while you're on meds. Again, that's not usually something to panic about. If it is orange or red, your doctor needs to know, as you may be bleeding. But if it's just a more intense yellow, it generally means that your body is flushing more solids, and that's a good thing. As your water intake increases, the intensity will subside. If you're changing your diet, that may also affect the color of urine. When we're ill, we tend to worry about a lot of things that just don't warrant it, and we sometimes imagine that things are far worse than they are.

Let your doctor know about anything that's abnormal,

and once that's done, don't let small concerns interfere with your day.

New shoes that are looser and have better insoles are a great idea for people with gout. Just one size wider can often help. Have your feet measured next time you're at the mall: most people's feet expand every year as they get older, and many of us are wearing shoes half a size too short and a couple of grades too narrow. If you work on concrete and stand all day, invest in cushioned mats for the floor around your workstation. Your boss may even want to contribute…

Coping with a gout attack also includes doing something that an alarming number of patients fail to do. Listen to your doctor. If he/she tells you to lay off the Alfredo sauce, then lay off the Alfredo sauce. Gout is one of the most common diseases in America, and the medical profession has been dealing with it for a very long time.

They know what they're talking about.

Chapter 5
Drug Therapies

Traditional Chinese doctors treat gout with herbs, a change in diet, and acupuncture. In Western medicine, we do two of those three things. We change our diet, and we use pharmaceuticals that are primarily plant-based. As the world shrinks, the two schools of thought seem to merge more and more. Western doctors who once dismissed acupuncture are now taking a serious look at the science behind it. One derivative of this more inclusive approach is that physical therapists are using directed electronic stimuli in much the same way that traditional Oriental doctors use needles.

For the time being, the most effective treatment for gout seems to be one set of drugs that quell attacks (usually NSAIDs: more on these in a minute), and another that helps prevent recurrences (most often, Allopurinol). The hard truth is that three out of four people who have a documented case of gout will end up having several more. Months and even years may pass before Round 2, but the odds are that gout will revisit.

Depending on the frequency of attacks, your doctor may or may not prescribe preventive medicine. If they occur once every two or three years, there doesn't seem to be much benefit from taking daily pills. If, however, they occur once a year or more frequently, then a daily medication that works on reducing uric acid levels is usually recommended.

Allopurinol

This drug is preventative, used to ward off future attacks rather than treat a current one. It reduces uric acid levels without producing too many detrimental side effects. If there is a reaction (and it's quite uncommon), it will most likely begin with a skin rash. If one appears within a week or two of starting Allopurinol, stop taking the pills and check with your doctor.

This is the best drug for anyone who has kidney problems, or kidney stones that were caused by high levels of uric acid. Unfortunately, this drug also has the potential to lower blood properties that help fight infections. And it can possibly reduce the ability to clot (making it easier to bleed). Because it works in the realm of the immune system, it may make you more susceptible to catching contagious diseases. Some marketers of Allopurinol state that it may impair your thinking or reactions. I haven't noticed that, although my family doesn't agree...

The drug company that makes my brand of allopurinol (and there are dozens) also warns about numerous other unlikely but still possible side effects, so a patient should read the paperwork from the pharmacy and also visit the drug maker's Web site before taking this or any drug.

Anecdotal evidence (that is, we have spoken with several gout sufferers who have been on Allopurinol for a decade or more) indicates that there are very few, if any, bad side effects for most people. What the drug does is reduce the level of an enzyme that creates uric acid. Unfortunately, in the process of doing this, it gets used up, so we have to continually repeat the dose. If we stop taking it, our bodies go right back to overproducing uric acid. It doesn't cure the reason we are producing so much acid, but it does prevent us suffering the results of long-term high levels of uric acid, such as joint damage and the emergence of tophi.

People who suffer repetitive attacks of gout should have their uric acid level tested regularly. Talk with your doctor about this.

For adults with gout, most doctors like to see a current attack completely abate, have the patient be totally devoid of symptoms for several days or even weeks, and then prescribe 200 to 300 mg orally once a day. In some cases of moderately severe gout where tophi are present, the dose is increased to 400 to 600 mg/day, which is administered in divided doses. Uric acid levels should begin to decline within a day or so, and the full effect is usually in place within a couple of weeks.

Allopurinol may react to several other drugs including but by no means limited to antibiotics (ampicillin and amoxicillin), blood thinners (dicoumarol or warfarin), and diuretic water pills. It can also help prevent a certain type of kidney stone that derives from acid crystals (but not all kidney stones).

The makers of Uloric®, a drug similar to allopurinol (but not a version of it), claim that the results of a recent study showed that "more patients with mild to moderate kidney problems reached a healthy uric acid level (less than 6 mg/dL) while taking ULORIC compared with allopurinol. Unlike patients using allopurinol, patients with mild to moderate kidney problems do not have to change doses with ULORIC. Only a small number of patients with severe kidney problems were studied. If you have kidney problems, ask your healthcare professional about the differences between medicines used to lower uric acid levels."

The Uloric Website is: www.uloric.com

NSAIDs

These are "nonsteroidal anti-inflammatory drugs", and they reduce the inflammation caused by those needle-like crystals that have accumulated in the joint. They are usually the first line of defense during an attack of gout. Some doctors will also recommend low doses of a NSAID on a daily basis, to prevent new flare-ups. The most common anti-inflammatory is Indomethacin.

The body makes a family of chemicals called prostaglandins, whose job is to do exactly what gout sufferers fear. They induce and develop inflammation, pain, and fever. They also help platelets form into blood clots, to stop us bleeding. And they defend the stomach lining from acid. For those with an interest in biology, prostaglandins are made by two cyclooxygenase enzymes called COX-1 and COX-2. Only COX-1 prostaglandins help platelets and defend the stomach.

NSAIDs block all of the good work done by prostaglandins and the result is that inflammation, pain, and fever can diminish. But the drugs also reduce the ability to clot, and because the stomach's defenses are reduced, they can cause ulcers and bleeding. If you have hemorrhoids, there's a chance that a high dose of indomethacin will make them bleed. If you have blood in your stool, immediately stop taking the drug and call your doctor.

NSAIDs can cause headaches.

Unless specifically directed by your doctor, NEVER take over-the-counter ibuprofen or similar drugs at the same time as a prescribed NSAID, as this will definitely increase the chance of bleeding.

Probenecid

This drug stops the body re-absorbing uric acid, which causes us to excrete more of it, which in turn reduces the volume of uric acid and thus its ability to crystallize. When first prescribed, it can actually increase uric acid levels, so doctors often prescribe colchicine or a NSAID too, at least for a few months. Patients taking Probenecid are generally instructed to drink two liters of fluid a day, to prevent kidney stones. People with kidney problems generally avoid this drug. Avoid aspirin when taking this drug, as it may block its effect on the kidneys.

Corticosteroid

Steroids were once thought to be the cure for arthritis. After World War II, they produced wonderful results, but their luster diminished as we discovered their side effects. Most obviously, sports personalities suffered infertility, brittle bones and a host of other problems related to them. Today, this family of powerful drugs can be quite valuable, as we now understand their effects and dosages. One treatment for gout is an injection of corticosteroid, which can often eradicate an attack in a matter of hours.

Colchicine

Not as dramatic as NSAIDs or steroid injections, this medicine has been used for more than two thousand years (that's not a typo) to treat gout. It is often prescribed for patients whose systems have problems handling NSAIDs. It used to be quite inexpensive, but in recent years the drug companies managed to increase the price to several dollars a pill. As I understand it, their argument seems to be that, after a couple of thousand years in use, it just hadn't been tested adequately in the field. Oh, well…

Colchicane suppresses inflammation. How it does that is apparently unknown, despite the price increase that paid for further study. Best guesses are that it helps to reduce the rate and/or volume of crystals being produced. While it's not in itself a painkiller, as it reduces inflammation the pain also decreases. Colchicane works best the sooner it is taken after an attack begins. It has been known to cause diarrhea, nausea, and abdominal cramping. It's not as popular as the NSAID drugs because it takes longer to work, and also in part because of the possible side effects, but it's gentler.

The way this drug works is that it blocks the early stages of inflammation, which explains why it should be used as early as possible. Unfortunately, it is less effective the longer one delays in starting it.

Other Drugs

In some cases, narcotic pain medication such as codeine and Demerol® are prescribed to reduce the pain of advanced gout.

Sulfinpyrazone, which lowers uric acid in the blood through excretion, is sometimes used to prevent future attacks. It has no beneficial effect on a current attack, but it can help dissolve tophi in advanced gout. Avoid aspirin when taking this drug, as it may block its effect on the kidneys.

Ask your doctor about baking soda. There is a school of thought that it can increase the alkalinity of urine, and reduce the risk of stones forming in the urinary tract.

Drugs work well, but your doctor will also ask you to lose weight, and do so slowly. You may also be advised to avoid red wines and beer, meat, fowl and seafoods, fat, asparagus, cauliflower, beans, peas, mushrooms, spinach and legumes.

Chapter 6
Exercise and Weight Control

This is the most painful part of the program for most of us – so painful, in fact, that we're actually willing to put up with gout rather than lose a few pounds.

That's just nuts.

And I'm the biggest nut.

Over the past three decades my weight has slowly crept from 170 lbs. to about 250 (I'm 6 foot 2 inches), and because the gain was incremental (only 3.5 ounces a month) it has never seemed dramatic. Unfortunately, the reverse is also true. Losing just a pound or two a month is such a small success that it's not quite dramatic enough to be rewarding. But even two pounds a month will eliminate all of that weight gain in a little over three years, and that's my plan. Slow, steady decline is exactly what's required. It's less traumatic on the body, and because it's the result of a small lifestyle change rather than a single dramatic gesture, it has a far higher chance of succeeding.

In 2005, Dr. Hyon Choi, a researcher at Massachusetts General Hospital, published a study in the *Archives of Internal Medicine*, which asserted that losing weight is the best way to prevent gout [9]. He and his research team established that overweight guys are gout victims waiting to happen. Among his findings was that "weight loss greater than 10 lbs. was associated with a substantially reduced risk of gout," and "men who had gained 30 lbs. or more had a twofold increased risk of gout compared with those who had maintained their weight."

One of the most startling findings of this study was that "in our cohort, 91% of gout cases occurred among men with a BMI of 23 or greater." In layman's terms that means, if you have a propensity toward gout, every extra pound you carry increases the odds of you having a lifetime of recurrent attacks.

After years of wimping out on weight-loss, I'm finally listening to my own doctor. All I do is eat a bit less at every meal, and stop eating between meals. For example, lunch nowadays is something like a mug of minestrone soup and some bread. In days past, I'd have had a sandwich with the soup, and maybe some chips, thereby adding hundreds of calories and lots of fat to the equation.

Switching from pop (soda) to water is a huge decision for most of us who lug around a few extra pounds. It reduces our risk for diabetes, knocks off the pounds, and increases our long-term energy level. If we make no other change than that, it probably will add years (and definitely healthier ones) to our lives. The way to make this change is to keep it up for only a week, and then for just one more week, until it becomes so ingrained that it's akin to the way that reformed smokers regard cigarettes. When we stay off pop long enough to lose the longing for it, we can actually start to dislike it. The thought of such a sweet, sugary drink becomes a little unpleasant.

I'm not an advocate of diet drinks and sugar substitutes, because of the chemicals involved. If you're giving up pop, the real dividends come if you can persuade yourself to settle for water, not diet drinks.

There is an eye-opening essay on this topic by Marcelle Pick on the Women To Women website:

www.womentowomen.com/healthyweight/splenda.aspx

The key to weight loss isn't fancy diets or expensive programs. It's having a goal for one day, or maybe for one week, and the goal needs to be behavioral, not quantitative. That is, we must decide to do, or not do, something specific for a certain time period. We must modify a behavior (I'll leave the chips on the plate, or only eat one half of the sandwich, or have water instead of pop) and put a limit on it (every day until Sunday). Quantitative goals (such as reaching a certain number of pounds lost by a certain date) simply don't work for most of us. They sound like they will, but they won't. Behavioral goals do work. They're immediate. The rewards are now. We can see and feel that we have changed something every time we do it. And so every time is a quiet, personal victory. We're not smart enough to fool ourselves, but we're reasonable enough to argue with ourselves.

What weight loss does for gout:
The first and most obvious benefit of weight loss is simply volume. If a 250 lb. guy works his way down to 190, he's going to produce less urine, and less uric acid. His body will also be running at a much better metabolic rate because it's only handling what it needs, rather than storing away all those extra calories as fat. All of the organs will be more effective, including the kidneys.

The next benefit is mechanical. Gout-susceptible ankle or toe joints that are supporting a 250 lb. mass have to work 24% more than those holding up a 190 lb. man. Think of bones, joints, cartilage and muscle as having been engineered to support you at your optimum weight. If you ask them to lift 124% of that every day, hour after hour, that's like driving your vehicle all the time in a lower gear that constantly ramps up the RPMs by 24%. If you did that, you'd expect some engine parts to fail.

The third benefit to weight loss is a bit subtle, but still very real. Overweight people are not as active as they should be. People who are slim tend to feel more like walking every day, and as they do, they get those synovial fluids in the joints moving. And that movement helps keep the crystals of uric acid from settling. Because the joints don't need to work as hard, they don't heat up as much. That means they don't spend a lot of the night recovering from stress and minor inflammation. Without inflammation, blood chemicals don't need to migrate there to fight imagined infection. All of this combined means that gout doesn't have as many invitations to visit during the night. No matter what way you slice it, losing weight slowly and steadily is a good idea.

BMI

So, what's an ideal weight? The scales are constantly changing because the "average" American is changing, too. We are, as a nation, becoming more obese and less active. We are also becoming a lot more ethnically diverse. Body Mass Index (BMI) is a number that is arrived at by combining a person's weight and height to see how much extra fat they are carrying.

To calculate your own BMI, you can visit the Centers for Disease Control and Prevention's website:

http://www.cdc.gov/healthyweight/assessing/bmi

Use the handy calculator there that's designed to destroy any illusions we may have about being fat. At 6 foot 2 inches and 250 lbs., I discovered to my horror that I was not only overweight, but actually obese (BMI 32.1). I need to get down to 233 lbs. just to be overweight (BMI 29.9), and hit 194 lbs. or less to be in my "normal" weight zone (BMI 24.9). Seeing it in black and white (well, in liquid crystal) is startling.

Alcohol and Gout

Gout sufferers need to watch their alcohol intake. One doesn't need to be a complete teetotaler, but there is a proven link between drinking and gout. Researchers at Massachusetts General list six triggers for gout, and the first one is booze: consumption of alcohol, consumption of protein-rich foods, fatigue, emotional stress, minor surgery and illness. A study that was published in the Canadian Medical Association's journal as far back as 1984 found that "a significant relation was found between alcohol abuse and acute gout" [10]. The Harvard Medical School maintains that "men who drink alcohol, particularly beer, may double their likelihood of developing gout" [11], and they back up this statement with research. "In a study published in *The Lancet* medical journal," the School's *Family Health Guide* says, "men who drank the most alcohol daily had twice the risk of developing the disorder as men who did not drink. Beer drinkers increased their risk by 50% for every daily serving, while those who drank hard liquor increased their risk by 15% for each drink."

There are two reasons to cut down on alcohol.

The first is that grain-based fluids usually have a high to very high purine content, which increases the level of uric acid in the blood. The second is that drinking packs on the pounds (lots of sugar), and overweight men are far more susceptible to gout. There is some research that suggests white wine doesn't incite an attack of gout, but red wine may. The results aren't definitive.

Chapter 7
A Good Gout Diet

The *New England Journal of Medicine* published a report in 2004 [12] that concluded: "Higher levels of meat and seafood consumption are associated with an increased risk of gout, whereas a higher level of consumption of dairy products is associated with a decreased risk. Moderate intake of purine-rich vegetables or protein is not associated with an increased risk of gout." (Note the word "moderate".)

While food in itself isn't the sole cause of gout, the purines in many of the foods that we eat can increase uric acid levels just enough to bring on gout. A sensible, low-purine diet, in conjunction with an exercise program (even just 30 minutes a day of walking) can dramatically reduce the chances of an attack.

The easiest way to stay on a low-purine diet is to bring a list to the supermarket that catalogs all of the good (low purine) ingredients that can be eaten, and also the bad (high purine) ones that should be avoided. If the fridge and kitchen cabinets only have good ingredients available, it's a lot easier to cook and eat right.

There are also a lot of foods that are somewhere in the middle. If you eat too much of these, they will be a problem. However, an occasional small helping isn't going to hurt too much.

Perhaps the biggest challenge is eating out. Restaurants can't possibly tell us all of the ingredients they're using. The best advice here is to avoid fast food completely, limit overall restaurant dining, and try to graze on the salad bar if possible (although some veggies are high purine foods, too). Soups and sauces are usually made with meat or poultry bases that are high in purines. Some fruits and veggies to avoid are bananas, broccoli, cauliflower, green peppers, peas, peanuts, spinach, and even tofu! Caffeine in soft drinks, tea and coffee can be a gout trigger, too.

The following lists of low, moderate and high purine foods are not exclusive, and in some cases there are differences of opinion among the experts as to which group certain foods belong (for example, alcoholic beverages). What we have done here is research as many reliable sources as possible, cross-reference the various lists, and come up with a sensible delineation. The idea is to use as many of the low purine ingredients as possible in daily use, dip into the moderate list every now and then, and if possible avoid the high purine foods. If the majority of your diet stays within these bounds, an occasional discretion most probably won't induce an attack of gout.

It's extremely important that you discuss any diet changes with your doctor, as he/she is concerned with your entire body, and not just your big toe. For example, nuts are low in purines, but if you have diverticulosis in your colon, they're probably not such a great idea. Diabetics, especially, should consult with their doctor before switching to a mainly fruit, pasta and vegetable diet. There's not much sense in managing gout, which isn't usually life threatening when treated with drug therapies, if the program gives another more dangerous disease a foothold.

Ask your doctor about monitoring your uric acid levels through blood tests. He/she may want to test you every six months or so, just to keep on top of things and see if the low-purine diet is doing its job. And don't assume that the diet replaces any drugs that your doctor has prescribed.

Low Purine Foods: Enjoy!

Blueberries
Bread - white/refined flour
Brown rice
Butter
Cabbage - red
Cake
Celery
Cereal
Cheese - low fat
Cherries - fresh
Chocolate
Cocoa
Cookies in small amounts
Cornbread
Crackers
Cream in moderation
Cream-style soups made with low-fat milk
Custard
Eggs in moderation
Fat-free dairy
Fats and oils in small amounts.
Fruit
Fruit juice
Gelatin
Herbs
Kale
Leafy green vegetables
Low-fat dairy products
Macaroni

Mandarin oranges

Margarine

Milk: skim or 1%

Noodles

Nuts

Oranges

Parsley

Pasta

Peanut butter

Peppers - red bell

Pickles

Pineapple

Popcorn

Potatoes

Pudding

Red cabbage

Relishes

Rice

Salt

Soups made without meat broth

Sugar

Syrup

Tangerines

Vegetables - except those listed

Vinegar

Water (8 glasses per day)

White bread

White sauce

Moderate Purine Foods: Occasional Use

Asparagus
Beef
Cantaloupe
Cauliflower
Chicken
Crab
Dried beans
Hazelnuts
Lamb
Lentils
Lobster
Marinated Green Olives
Oats and oatmeal
Oysters
Pork
Shrimp
Spinach
Strawberries
Tomato
Tuna fish in water
Watercress
Wheat germ and bran
Whole wheat bread

High Purine Foods: Avoid These

Alcoholic

Anchovies

Apple

Aubergine

Bacon

Bananas

Beans

Beef kidneys

Beer

Bouillon

Brains

Broccoli

Broth

Brussels Sprouts

Cabbage - white/green

Carrots

Caviar

Chicory

Cod

Consommé

Cucumbers

Duck

Figs, dried

Fish roe

Foie Gras

Game meats

Goose

Grapes

Gravy

Green peas
Green peppers
Grouse
Haddock
Hearts
Herring
Kidneys
Kiwi fruit
Leeks
Lettuce
Liver
Lunchmeats
Mackerel
Meat extracts
Mincemeat
Mushrooms
Mussels
Mutton
Organ meats
Partridge
Pheasant
Red meat
Rhubarb
Roe (fish eggs)
Salmon
Sardines
Scallops
Smelt
Soya beans
Sweetbreads

Trout
Tuna fish in oil
Turkey
Veal
Venison
Yeast
Yeast supplements

These lists are not exclusive. As new studies emerge, the recommendations tend to change because medical opinions become more informed.

You may want to take this book with you when grocery shopping.

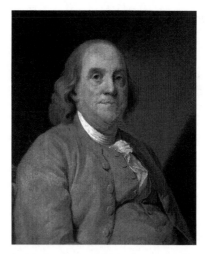

Benjamin Franklin suffered terribly from gout.

Sources

1 http://www.health.harvard.edu/fhg/updates/Gout-Joint-pain-and-more.shtml
2 http://www.nlm.nih.gov/medlineplus/ency/article/003476.htm
3 http://www.mayoclinic.com/health/high-uric-acid-
level/MY00160/DSECTION=causes
4 http://www.elsevier.com/wps/find/bookdescription.cws_home/716563/description
5 http://www.whfoods.com/genpage.php?tname=george&dbid=51
6 http://www.footdoc.ca/www.FootDoc.ca/Website%20Gout.htm
7 http://www.arthritistoday.org/conditions/gout/all-about-gout/gout-triggers.php
8 http://health.nytimes.com/health/guides/disease/gout-chronic/triggers.html
9 http://archinte.ama-assn.org/cgi/content/full/165/7/742
10 http://www.cmaj.ca/content/131/6/563.abstract?sid=55e82cbd-7ccf-46cf-817b-
4a2659fbbbba
11 http://www.health.harvard.edu/fhg/updates/update0804a.shtml
12 http://www.nejm.org/doi/full/10.1056/NEJMoa035700

The **Arthritis Foundation** has a very helpful page
on their site for gout patients, which is located at:

http://www.arthritis.org/goutliving.php

The Foundation funds lots of research and disseminates
a great deal of information. It's also one of the places that
doctors can visit to catch up on the latest studies, news, and
drug therapies.
To support the Foundation's ongoing research (and
your help is truly needed), please go to www.arthritis.org
and click on DONATE. The author has no connection
whatsoever to the Foundation.

Made in the USA
Middletown, DE
06 June 2021